Morning Face Treatment Essentials

Harmonizing Mind, Body, and Skin in your Daily Routine for a Lasting Glow

Larry A. Harris

Dedication

To the unwavering support and boundless love of my parents who have been the steadfast pillars upon which my dreams have soared. Your encouragement and belief in my journey have been the driving force behind every word penned in this book.

To my well-wishers, whose optimism and cheering voices have echoed in the background of my writing days, providing the motivation needed to overcome challenges and embrace triumphs. Your belief in my creative endeavors has been a source of inspiration that I carry with pride.

And, above all, to the Almighty, the Divine orchestrator of destinies, who granted me the gift of creativity and the opportunity to weave stories. In moments of solitude and uncertainty, your guidance has been my compass, steering me through the labyrinth of imagination.

May the words within these pages be a humble offering of gratitude to those whose love and blessings have illuminated my path. This book is dedicated to the enduring spirits of family, friendship, and the Divine forces that shape our narratives.

Table of Contents

Introduction: Brief Overview

In the hustle and bustle of modern life, a night of restful sleep is considered a luxury. However, for those who wake up to find imprints and lines etched onto their faces, sleep becomes a fascinating puzzle to solve. This phenomenon, commonly known as "morning pillow prints," is more than just a temporary inconvenience; it's a silent messenger from our skin, revealing insights into our health and skin-care habits.

This book aims to unravel the mysteries behind those pillow prints that greet us in the mirror each morning. From the science behind their formation to the messages they convey about our skin, we will embark on a journey to understand the subtle language spoken by these creases. Beyond a mere aesthetic concern, pillow prints can be indicative of underlying issues that merit attention.

Importance of Morning Pillow Prints

While pillow prints might be dismissed as a byproduct of a restless night or an uncomfortable pillow, their significance goes beyond the surface. These morning creases act as mirrors reflecting the health and condition of our skin. Understanding their implications can empower us to take proactive steps in our skin-care routine and overall wellbeing.

Imagine waking up to a canvas imprinted with fine lines and wrinkles – the skin's way of whispering about its hydration needs and elasticity. These imprints aren't just temporary blemishes; they are messages begging for attention. The importance of recognizing and interpreting these signs cannot be overstated. In a world where the skin-care industry bombards us with endless products and routines, our own skin has a story to tell, etched in the lines that appear while we slumber.

Furthermore, the study of morning pillow prints provides a unique perspective on the science of sleep. Our sleep positions, pillow materials, and even the quality of our bedding play a crucial role in the development of these facial imprints. By delving into the intricacies of this nocturnal phenomenon, we gain insights that extend beyond skin-care, offering a holistic view of how our nightly routines impact our waking hours.

Chapter 1: The Science Behind Pillow Prints

Understanding the Causes

1. Pressure Points: Mapping the Contact Zones:

Pillow prints, those temporary imprints left on your face after a night's sleep, are a fascinating phenomenon that often provides clues about the science of sleep and skin health. One of the primary causes of pillow prints lies in the distribution of pressure points as you rest your head on a pillow.

Anatomy of Pressure Points:

Forehead: The area around the forehead, especially where the head rests, is susceptible to pressure points.

Cheeks: Cheekbones and the sides of the face bear the weight of the head, leading to indentations.

Nose and Mouth: The bridge of the nose and the area around the mouth may also develop pillow prints due to sustained pressure.

Blood Flow and Pressure:

As you sleep, blood flow to certain areas of the face may be restricted, causing temporary changes in skin texture.

Pressure points can affect circulation, leading to reduced oxygen and nutrient delivery to the skin.

Impact on Skin Health:

Prolonged pressure on specific areas can contribute to the development of fine lines and wrinkles over time.

Understanding the science behind pressure points allows for targeted prevention and skin-care strategies.

2. Sleep Positions: Unveiling the Influence on Pillow Prints:

The way you position your head and face on the pillow has a significant impact on the formation of pillow prints. Different sleep positions can create unique patterns of pressure and indentation.

Back Sleeping:

Back sleepers may notice pillow prints primarily on the forehead and the back of the head.

The pressure is distributed more evenly, reducing the likelihood of deep imprints.

Side Sleeping:

Side sleepers often experience pillow prints on one side of the face, including the cheek and jawline.

The pillow compresses the skin against the underlying bone structure, leaving distinct marks.

Stomach Sleeping:

Stomach sleepers may develop pillow prints on the forehead and one side of the face.

This position can create more pronounced lines due to sustained pressure on specific areas.

Impact on Facial Contours:

The repeated compression of the skin against the pillow can influence the development of lines and wrinkles.

Sleep positions contribute to the overall texture and appearance of facial contours.

How Pillow Prints Develop

1.   The Role of Collagen and Elasticity:

Understanding how pillow prints develop involves delving into the skin's structure and the role of key components like collagen and elastin.

Collagen's Supportive Matrix:

Collagen provides structural support to the skin, forming a matrix that maintains its firmness and resilience.

Over time, factors like pressure and sleep positions can affect collagen fibers, leading to the formation of creases.

Elasticity and Skin Rebound:

Elastin contributes to skin elasticity, allowing it to stretch and rebound.

Pillow prints reveal insights into the skin's elasticity and its ability to recover from external pressure.

2. Dehydration and Pillow Prints: Unveiling the Connection:

Dehydration is a significant factor that can intensify the development of pillow prints. The skin's hydration levels influence its pliability and susceptibility to compression.

How Dehydration Affects the Skin:

Dehydrated skin lacks the necessary moisture to maintain its suppleness.

When the skin is dehydrated, it becomes more prone to developing visible lines and imprints.

Preventing DehydrationRelated Pillow Prints:

Hydrating the skin through a wellrounded skin-care routine can mitigate the impact of dehydration on the development of pillow prints.

Using moisturizers with hydrating ingredients contributes to the skin's overall resilience.

3. Sleep Environment and Pillow Fabric: Influencers of Pillow Prints:

Beyond individual factors, the sleep environment and the choice of pillow fabric also play a role in the development of pillow prints.

Pillow Fabric and Friction:

The type of pillowcase fabric can affect friction against the skin.

Silk or satin pillowcases, for example, may cause less friction compared to cotton, potentially reducing the intensity of pillow prints.

Thread Count and Smoothness:

Higher thread count in pillowcases often results in a smoother surface.

A smoother surface can reduce the likelihood of deep imprints, especially for those with sensitive or easily creased skin.

Temperature and Humidity:

Extreme temperatures and low humidity can contribute to skin dryness, making it more susceptible to pressureinduced imprints.

Maintaining a comfortable sleep environment with optimal temperature and humidity levels supports skin health.

Mitigating Pillow Prints: Strategies for Prevention

1. Choosing the Right Pillow:

Selecting the right pillow can make a significant difference in mitigating the development of pillow prints. Consider factors such as pillow type, loft, and material.

Memory Foam Pillows:

Memory foam pillows conform to the shape of your head and neck, providing even support and reducing pressure points.

Opting for a memory foam pillow can contribute to minimizing the intensity of pillow prints.

Adjustable Loft Pillows:

Pillows with adjustable loft allow you to customize the height based on your sleep position.

Proper neck support helps distribute pressure more evenly, reducing the likelihood of pronounced pillow prints.

Silk or Satin Pillowcases:

Smooth and silky pillowcases reduce friction against the skin, contributing to a gentler sleeping surface.

Silk or satin pillowcases can be particularly beneficial for those prone to developing deep imprints.

2. Incorporating skin-care into Your Evening Routine:

Your evening skin-care routine can play a crucial role in preparing your skin for a restful night's sleep.

Hydrating Products:

Use hydrating products such as moisturizers and serums in your evening routine to boost skin hydration.

Wellhydrated skin is less prone to developing deep imprints.

Avoiding Harsh Ingredients:

Be mindful of skin-care products containing harsh ingredients that may increase skin sensitivity.

Opt for gentle formulations to minimize the risk of irritation and inflammation.

Consistent skin-care Practices:

Consistency in your skin-care routine helps maintain skin health and resilience.

A well-maintained skin barrier is better equipped to handle external pressures during sleep.

3. Changing Sleep Positions: A Conscious Shift:

While changing one's preferred sleep position may not be easy, making gradual adjustments can positively impact the development of pillow prints.

Back Sleeping Strategies:

Placing a small pillow under the knees can encourage back sleeping by providing additional comfort.

Back sleeping distributes pressure more evenly, reducing the likelihood of deep imprints.

Side Sleeping Modifications:

Using a body pillow for support can help maintain a more neutral spine alignment.

Adjusting pillow height can minimize pressure on the cheek and jawline for side sleepers.

Stomach Sleeping Considerations:

Stomach sleeping is often associated with a higher risk of developing pronounced pillow prints.

Gradually transitioning to side or back sleeping can be beneficial for skin health.

4. Silk or Satin Sleep Accessories: A Luxurious Solution:

Embracing silk or satin sleep accessories goes beyond pillowcases and can extend to sleep masks and hair wraps.

Benefits of Silk Sleep Accessories:

Silk or satin sleep accessories reduce friction against the skin, contributing to a smoother sleep experience.

These materials are gentle on the hair, reducing the risk of morning hair creases.

5. DIY Remedies for Morning Skin Revitalization:

Incorporating DIY remedies into your morning routine can help revitalize the skin and reduce the visibility of pillow prints.

Facial Massage:

Gently massaging the face in the morning promotes blood circulation and helps reduce puffiness.

Focus on areas with visible pillow prints to encourage skin recovery.

Cool Compress:

Applying a cool compress to the face can help soothe the skin and minimize morning puffiness.

This simple remedy can enhance the overall appearance of the skin.

Hydrating Mist:

A hydrating mist with ingredients like aloe vera or rosewater can refresh the skin and provide an instant boost of hydration.

Spritzing the mist on areas with pillow prints contributes to skin revitalization.

Pillow prints, while temporary and harmless, offer a unique window into the dynamic relationship between sleep, skin-care, and skin health. Understanding the science behind pillow prints empowers individuals to make informed choices about their sleep environment, skin-care routine, and lifestyle.

As we navigate the intricate interplay of pressure points, sleep positions, and skin biology, it becomes clear that mitigating pillow prints involves a holistic approach. From selecting the right pillow and adjusting sleep positions to incorporating skin-care practices and DIY remedies, individuals can actively participate in preserving the youthful and resilient quality of their skin.

Chapter 2: Decoding Pillow Prints

Different Types of Pillow Prints

1. Lines and Wrinkles: Insights into Aging and Sleep Habits:

Pillow prints come in various forms, each offering insights into both aging processes and sleep habits. Lines and wrinkles are among the most common types of pillow prints, and their appearance can reveal valuable information about the skin's elasticity and how it responds to pressure.

Expression Lines:

Pillow prints resembling fine lines may indicate the presence of expression lines on the face.

These lines, often associated with facial expressions, can become more prominent with age and extended periods of pressure during sleep.

Sleep Creases and Skin Aging:

Wrinkles and creases that persist after waking up may be indicative of the skin's aging process.

Reduced collagen and elastin levels contribute to the formation of wrinkles, and the pressure exerted during sleep can accentuate their appearance.

Preventing SleepInduced Wrinkles:

Using antiaging skin-care products, such as those containing retinoids, can help minimize the impact of sleepinduced wrinkles.

Adjusting sleep positions to reduce facial pressure points can contribute to wrinkle prevention.

2. Imprints and Indentations: The Canvas of Sleep Patterns:

Imprints and indentations left by the pillow on the face are like a canvas that reflects the unique sleep patterns and preferences of individuals. These distinctive marks offer a visual record of how sleep positions influence the skin's surface.

Side Sleeper's Indentations:

Side sleepers often experience imprints on one side of the face, corresponding to the pillow's compression against the cheek and jawline.

These indentations provide a snapshot of the preferred sleep position and the associated pressure points.

Forehead Imprints and Sleep Positions:

Forehead imprints may indicate pressure points resulting from back or stomach sleeping positions.

The specific location of imprints helps identify the predominant areas of facial contact with the pillow.

Duration of Imprints: Insights into Sleep Quality:

The duration and depth of pillow imprints can offer insights into the overall sleep quality.

Deeper imprints may suggest longer periods of sustained pressure, potentially impacting skin health.

The Intersection of Pillow Prints and Skin Health

1. Pillow Prints as a Reflection of Skin Resilience:

The presence and characteristics of pillow prints serve as a visual reflection of the skin's resilience and ability to rebound from external pressures. Understanding this intersection provides a deeper appreciation for the dynamic relationship between sleep and skin health.

Skin Resilience and Elasticity:

Pillow prints that fade quickly after waking up may indicate good skin resilience and elasticity.

A skinfriendly pillowcase and wellhydrated skin contribute to the ability of the skin to bounce back from compression.

Persistent Imprints and Skin Sensitivity:

Imprints that linger for an extended period may suggest heightened skin sensitivity.

Individuals with sensitive skin may experience more pronounced reactions to pressure, necessitating gentle skin-care practices.

2. Pillow Prints as Diagnostic Tools: Unveiling Potential Concerns:

While pillow prints are typically harmless and temporary, their characteristics can occasionally serve as diagnostic tools, unveiling potential concerns related to skin health and overall wellbeing.

Dehydration Indicators:

Pillow prints that appear more defined or pronounced may indicate dehydration.

Dehydrated skin lacks the necessary moisture to maintain its pliability, making it more susceptible to pressureinduced imprints.

Potential Circulation Issues:

Persistent pillow prints that are accompanied by redness or discoloration may warrant attention to potential circulation issues.

Restricted blood flow to certain areas during sleep can contribute to the development of visible imprints.

Skin Conditions and Pillow Prints:

Individuals with certain skin conditions, such as eczema or psoriasis, may notice unique patterns in their pillow prints. Understanding how specific skin conditions interact with sleep patterns can aid in managing symptoms.

Strategies for Decoding and Responding to Pillow Prints

1. Analyzing Pillow Prints for Sleep Improvement:

Decoding pillow prints involves not only understanding their visual cues but also using this information to make positive changes to sleep habits.

Identifying Preferred Sleep Positions:

Analyzing the location and depth of pillow prints helps identify preferred sleep positions.

Adjusting pillows and sleep positions to reduce pressure on specific areas can lead to more comfortable and beneficial sleep.

Experimenting with Pillow Types:
Trying different types of pillows, such as memory foam or adjustable loft pillows, allows individuals to find the most supportive option.

The right pillow can minimize pressure points and contribute to a more harmonious sleep experience.

2.   Tailoring skin-care to Pillow Print Patterns:
Tailoring skin-care routines to pillow print patterns involves acknowledging the areas of the face most affected by pressure and adapting skin-care practices accordingly.

Targeted skin-care Products:

Using targeted skin-care products, such as those addressing specific areas of concern highlighted by pillow prints, enhances the effectiveness of the routine.

For example, incorporating eye creams for undereye imprints or forehead-focused treatments for lines in those areas.

Consistent Hydration Practices:

Prioritizing consistent hydration through moisturizers and serums supports the overall health of the skin.

Wellhydrated skin is more resilient and less prone to the development of pronounced pillow prints.

3. Addressing Potential Underlying Issues:

While pillow prints are generally benign, addressing potential underlying issues revealed by persistent or unusual imprints is crucial for overall wellbeing.

Consulting with Dermatologists:

If pillow prints are accompanied by persistent redness, discomfort, or other concerning symptoms, consulting with a dermatologist is advisable.

Dermatologists can provide insights into potential skin conditions and recommend appropriate interventions.

Monitoring Changes Over Time:

Regularly monitoring changes in the characteristics of pillow prints over time helps individuals stay attuned to shifts in skin health.

Being proactive about adjustments to sleep habits and skin-care practices promotes longterm skin wellbeing.

Pillow Prints as Markers of Personal Wellness

1. Embracing the Uniqueness of Pillow Prints:

Pillow prints, far from being mere imprints on the face, serve as markers of personal wellness, reflecting the intricacies of sleep, skin-care, and individual habits.

Celebrating Individual Sleep Patterns:

Each person's pillow prints are a unique record of their sleep preferences and positions.

Embracing these patterns contributes to a deeper understanding of one's personal sleep journey.

Emphasizing Overall WellBeing:

Pillow prints go beyond skin-care; they are indicators of overall wellbeing.

Prioritizing good sleep hygiene, skin-care practices, and selfcare contributes to a holistic approach to health.

2. Promoting Positive Sleep Practices:

Decoding pillow prints encourages the promotion of positive sleep practices that benefit both the skin and overall health.

Creating a Comfortable Sleep Environment:

Investing in a comfortable mattress, pillows, and bedding enhances the sleep environment.

A conducive sleep environment minimizes pressure points and promotes restful sleep.

Establishing Consistent Sleep Routines:

Consistent sleep routines, including regular bedtimes and wakeup times, contribute to better sleep quality.

Wellregulated sleep patterns reduce the likelihood of pronounced pillow prints.

Pillow prints, with their diverse forms and patterns, tell a story—a story of sleep, skin-care, and the unique journey of each individual. As we decode the language of lines, wrinkles, imprints, and indentations, we gain insights into the dynamic relationship between external pressures and the skin's response.

Chapter 3: What Your Pillow Prints Are Trying to Tell You

Skin Health Indicator

Pillow prints, those temporary imprints left on your face after a night's sleep, are not just fleeting marks; they can be powerful indicators of your skin's health. Understanding what your pillow prints are trying to tell you provides valuable insights into potential issues and allows for targeted interventions to enhance your skin's wellbeing.

1. Dehydration: The Silent Culprit Behind Pronounced Pillow Prints:

Dehydration, a common skin concern, often leaves its mark in the form of pronounced pillow prints. These imprints can be more than just aesthetic—they might be signaling a need for increased hydration in your skin-care routine.

How Dehydration Manifests in Pillow Prints:

Dehydrated skin lacks the necessary moisture to maintain its suppleness.

Pillow prints on dehydrated skin tend to be more defined, reflecting the skin's reduced ability to bounce back from pressure.

Addressing Dehydration with skin-care:

Incorporating hydrating products into your skin-care routine helps replenish moisture.

Look for ingredients like hyaluronic acid, glycerin, and ceramides, which attract and retain water in the skin.

Hydration Beyond skin-care:

Hydration is not only about topical products; it's also influenced by internal factors.

Drinking an adequate amount of water and maintaining a balanced diet contribute to overall skin hydration.

Observing Changes in Pillow Print Intensity:

Monitoring changes in the intensity of pillow prints over time can indicate the effectiveness of hydrationfocused interventions.

A gradual reduction in pronounced imprints suggests improved skin hydration.

2. Lack of Moisture: Pillow Prints as Signals of Thirsty Skin:

Pillow prints that linger for an extended period or appear deeper than usual may be signaling a lack of moisture in the skin. This goes beyond dehydration and highlights the importance of maintaining a wellhydrated and moisturized skin barrier.

The Role of Moisturizers in Skin Health:

Moisturizers play a crucial role in sealing in hydration and preventing water loss from the skin.

Using a moisturizer tailored to your skin type ensures that your skin retains essential moisture.

Choosing the Right Moisturizer:

Individuals with dry skin benefit from richer, more emollient moisturizers.

For those with oily or combination skin, lightweight, noncomedogenic options are preferable.

Nighttime Moisturizing for Pillow Print Prevention:

Applying a hydrating night cream or sleeping mask before bedtime boosts overnight hydration.

Well-moisturized skin is less susceptible to developing deep pillow prints.

Personalizing Moisturization Strategies:

Tailoring your moisturization strategies based on seasonal changes and skin responses ensures continuous skin health.

Adjusting your routine to provide extra moisture during drier seasons contributes to optimal skin balance.

3. Allergies or Sensitivities: Pillow Prints as Sensitive Skin Signals:

Pillow prints that are accompanied by redness, itching, or irritation may indicate underlying allergies or sensitivities. The skin's reaction to certain materials or ingredients in skin-care products can manifest in visible imprints and discomfort.

Identifying Allergens in Bedding:

Pillowcase fabrics and laundry detergents may contain allergens that irritate the skin.

Opting for hypoallergenic bedding materials and fragrancefree detergents can minimize potential triggers.

Avoiding skin-care Ingredients That Cause Sensitivity:

Certain skin-care ingredients, such as fragrances and harsh chemicals, can exacerbate skin sensitivity.

Choosing skin-care products with gentle formulations reduces the risk of allergic reactions and irritation.

Patch Testing New Products: A Preemptive Approach:

Before introducing new skin-care products, conducting patch tests on a small area of skin helps identify potential allergies.

Patch testing minimizes the risk of widespread irritation, ensuring the compatibility of products with your skin.

Seeking Professional Guidance for Persistent Sensitivities:

If pillow prints are consistently accompanied by skin sensitivities, consulting with a dermatologist is advisable.

Dermatologists can perform allergy tests and recommend suitable skin-care products for sensitive skin.

Pillow Prints as Diagnostic Tools

1. Deeper Insights Through Persistent Pillow Prints:

While transient pillow prints are a natural part of waking up, persistent imprints that endure throughout the day may be trying to communicate more specific messages about your skin's condition.

Persistent Imprints and Circulation Issues:

Pillow prints that linger for an extended period and are accompanied by redness may indicate potential circulation issues.

Restricted blood flow during sleep can contribute to the development of more pronounced and persistent imprints.

Consulting with Healthcare Professionals:

If persistent pillow prints are a cause for concern, consulting with healthcare professionals, including dermatologists and vascular specialists, can provide a comprehensive evaluation.

Identifying and addressing underlying circulation issues is crucial for overall skin health.

2. Tracking Changes Over Time: A Dynamic Approach:

The characteristics of pillow prints can evolve over time, offering a dynamic snapshot of changes in your skin health. Regularly tracking these changes provides a proactive approach to skin-care.

Documenting Skin Responses:

Keeping a skin-care journal or documenting changes in pillow prints over time helps identify patterns and potential triggers.

This proactive approach allows for timely adjustments to skin-care routines.

Adapting skin-care Practices:

Adjusting skin-care practices based on observed changes ensures a personalized and evolving approach.

Periodic reassessment and adaptation contribute to ongoing skin health.

Collaborating with skin-care Professionals:

skin-care professionals, including dermatologists and aestheticians, can provide guidance on adapting skin-care routines.

Collaborating with professionals ensures evidencebased interventions tailored to individual skin needs.

Strategies for Pillow Print Prevention and Skin Health

1. Holistic Approaches to Pillow Print Prevention:

Preventing pillow prints goes beyond skin-care; it involves adopting holistic approaches that address both external and internal factors influencing skin health.

Optimizing Sleep Positions:

Experimenting with different sleep positions to minimize pressure points helps prevent pronounced pillow prints.

Back sleeping and using supportive pillows contribute to even pressure distribution.

Investing in Quality Bedding:

Choosing pillowcases made from smooth and gentle fabrics, such as silk or satin, reduces friction against the skin.

Investing in highquality bedding materials supports overall skin health.

Regulating Sleep Environment:

Maintaining a comfortable sleep environment with optimal temperature and humidity levels supports skin hydration.

Consistent sleep routines contribute to overall wellbeing, influencing the appearance of pillow prints.

2. Integrating DIY Remedies into Morning Rituals:

DIY remedies can play a role in revitalizing the skin and minimizing the visibility of pillow prints. Simple practices incorporated into your morning routine contribute to skin revitalization.

Facial Exercises for Improved Circulation:

Gentle facial exercises, such as facial massage and yoga, promote blood circulation.

Improved circulation contributes to faster skin recovery and reduced puffiness.

Cool Compress for Soothing the Skin:

Applying a cool compress to the face in the morning helps soothe the skin and minimize morning puffiness.

This DIY remedy enhances the overall appearance of the skin.

Hydrating Mists for Instant Refreshment:

Hydrating mists with ingredients like aloe vera or rosewater provide an instant boost of hydration.

Spritzing the mist on areas with pillow prints contributes to skin revitalization.

3. Customized skin-care Plans:

Professional Guidance for Optimal Skin Health:

Seeking professional guidance ensures that skin-care plans are tailored to individual skin types, concerns, and goals. Dermatologist visits and customized skin-care plans contribute to a comprehensive and effective approach. Dermatologist Visits for Skin Evaluation:

Regular dermatologist visits allow for professional evaluation of skin health.

Dermatologists can identify potential issues and recommend appropriate interventions.

Customized skin-care Plans: Addressing Unique Skin Needs:

Customized skin-care plans take into account individual skin needs and concerns.

Tailored recommendations enhance the effectiveness of skin-care routines.

Periodic Reassessment for Evolving Needs:

Periodic reassessment with skin-care professionals ensures that skin-care plans evolve with changing skin needs. Collaborating with professionals contributes to a proactive and personalized skin-care journey.

Pillow prints, those silent messengers on your face each morning, tell a nuanced story of your skin's health and wellbeing. From signals of dehydration and lack of moisture to potential allergies and sensitivities, these imprints provide a canvas for understanding and addressing skin concerns.

Chapter 4: Assessing Your Morning Skin

Self-Examination Techniques

The mirror serves as a portal into the intricate landscape of your skin, revealing the story written in the language of morning pillow prints. Assessing your morning skin involves more than a cursory glance; it requires a thoughtful examination that unveils the nuances of your skin's health and wellbeing. In this chapter, we will explore selfexamination techniques designed to empower you with the knowledge needed to decode the messages whispered by your pillow prints.

1. Lighting Matters:

Begin your examination in welllit surroundings. Natural daylight is ideal, providing a clear and accurate view of your skin. Avoid harsh, direct lighting, as it may cast shadows that obscure finer details. A softly illuminated room allows you to observe subtle changes, lines, and textures with precision.

2. Cleanse and Moisturize:

Before the examination, ensure your face is clean and free of makeup or skin-care products from the previous night. Gently cleanse your skin to remove any residues that might interfere with your observations. After cleansing, apply a light moisturizer to create a smooth canvas for assessment.

3. Observe Different Areas:

Your face is not a uniform canvas, and different areas may reveal distinct information. Pay attention to the forehead, eyes, cheeks, and mouth separately. Note the presence and characteristics of lines, wrinkles, or imprints in each region. Understanding variations across facial zones provides a comprehensive overview of your skin's condition.

4. Texture and Elasticity:

Use your fingertips to lightly touch different areas of your face. Assess the texture and elasticity of your skin. Does it feel dry, taut, or supple? Note any variations in texture, as it may indicate areas that require additional attention in your skin-care routine.

5. Expression and Relaxation:

Experiment with facial expressions during the examination. Smile, frown, and raise your eyebrows to observe how your skin responds. Pay attention to how quickly your skin returns to its neutral state after expressions. This dynamic assessment provides insights into your skin's flexibility and resilience.

6.   Understand Your Sleep Positions:

Reflect on your preferred sleep positions and how they might contribute to specific pillow prints. If you notice consistent imprints or lines on one side of your face, it could be linked to your habitual sleep position. Understanding these patterns allows you to make informed adjustments to minimize pressure points.

7. Evaluate Changes Over Time:

Regularly assess your morning skin and document any noticeable changes over time. This ongoing selfexamination enables you to track the effectiveness of skin-care adjustments, lifestyle changes, or new products. By identifying trends, you can refine your routine to better address the evolving needs of your skin.

By incorporating these selfexamination techniques into your morning routine, you transform your mirror into a valuable tool for understanding and nurturing your skin. The observations you make during this selfassessment serve as a foundation for informed decisionmaking, guiding your skin-care choices and routine adjustments.

Keeping a Pillow Print Journal

Your journey to healthier skin involves not only selfexamination but also the art of mindful observation. Keeping a Pillow Print Journal is a transformative practice that allows you to document the unique language spoken by your morning pillow prints. This journal becomes a chronicle of your skin's evolution, offering valuable insights into the effectiveness of your skin-care regimen and lifestyle choices.

1. Select a Dedicated Journal:

Choose a journal specifically for recording your pillow print observations. This could be a physical notebook or a digital journal based on your preference. Having a dedicated space ensures that you can easily reference and compare entries over time.

2. Establish a Routine:

Integrate the journaling practice into your morning routine. After completing your selfexamination, take a few minutes to record your observations. Establishing a consistent routine makes journaling a seamless and sustainable part of your daily habits.

3. Record Specifics:

Document specific details related to your morning pillow prints. Include information about the types of imprints, their intensity, and any changes you notice in comparison to previous entries. Note the products used the night before, your sleep position, and other relevant factors.

4.   Describe   Your   skin-care Routine:

Detail your skin-care routine leading up to the observed pillow prints. Include the products applied, their order, and any adjustments made to your routine. This documentation allows you to correlate specific skin-care practices with the resulting impact on your skin.

5. Note Lifestyle Factors:

Consider factors beyond skin-care, such as hydration, diet, and stress levels. Changes in these lifestyle factors can influence the appearance of your skin. By recording these elements in your journal, you gain a holistic understanding of how various aspects of your life contribute to your skin's health.

6. Reflect on Trends:

Periodically review your journal entries to identify patterns and trends. Look for correlations between certain skin-care products, sleep positions, or lifestyle choices and the observed changes in your skin. This reflective practice guides you in refining your approach for optimal skin health.

7. Celebrate Progress:

Acknowledge and celebrate positive changes in your skin. If adjustments to your routine lead to improvements, document these successes. Recognizing progress fosters a positive mindset and motivates continued commitment to your skin-care journey.

8. Adapt and Adjust:

Your Pillow Print Journal is a dynamic tool that evolves with your skin-care journey. Use it as a guide for adapting and adjusting your routine based on the insights gained. Embrace the flexibility to experiment with new products or habits while closely monitoring their impact.

In essence, a Pillow Print Journal is not merely a record of marks on your face; it is a narrative of your skin's responses, needs, and triumphs. This practice transforms the routine observation of pillow prints into a purposeful and empowering journey toward healthier, more radiant skin.

Chapter 5: Upgrading Your skin-care Routine

A well-crafted skin-care routine is the foundation of healthy, radiant skin. In this chapter, we will explore the art of upgrading your skin-care routine, focusing on the importance of choosing the right products and establishing a morning skin-care routine. Whether you're a skin-care enthusiast or a newcomer to the world of skin-care, the following insights will guide you in optimizing your routine for the best possible outcomes.

Choosing the Right Products

1.   Moisturizers: The Key to Hydration:

Moisturizers play a pivotal role in maintaining skin health by preventing dehydration, improving skin texture, and supporting the skin's natural barrier function. Choosing the right moisturizer involves considering your skin type, specific concerns, and desired outcomes.

For Dry Skin: Opt for rich, hydrating moisturizers that contain ingredients like hyaluronic acid, glycerin, and ceramides. These ingredients help replenish moisture and restore the skin's natural lipid barrier.

For Oily or AcneProne Skin: Look for noncomedogenic, oilfree formulas. Gelbased moisturizers with ingredients like niacinamide can provide hydration without clogging pores.

For Sensitive Skin: Choose fragrancefree and hypoallergenic moisturizers with calming ingredients such as chamomile or aloe vera. Avoid products with potential irritants like alcohol or synthetic fragrances.

For Combination Skin: Consider using different moisturizers for different areas of your face. For example, a lighter formula for the Tzone and a more hydrating one for drier areas.

2. AntiAging Products: Defying Time Gracefully:

Antiaging products are designed to address and prevent signs of aging, such as fine lines, wrinkles, and loss of elasticity. Incorporating these products into your skin-care routine is a proactive step toward maintaining youthful and vibrant skin.

Retinoids (Retinol, Tretinoin): Retinoids are powerful derivatives of vitamin A known for their ability to stimulate collagen production and promote cell turnover. They can diminish the appearance of fine lines, improve skin texture, and enhance overall radiance. Start with lower concentrations, especially if you have sensitive skin, and gradually increase over time.

Vitamin C Serums: Vitamin C is a potent antioxidant that helps neutralize free radicals, reduce hyperpigmentation, and boost collagen production. Incorporating a vitamin C serum into your routine can contribute to a brighter complexion and protect your skin from environmental damage.

Peptides: Peptides are amino acid compounds that support collagen synthesis and improve skin elasticity. Peptide-infused products can target specific aging concerns and enhance the overall firmness of your skin.

Hyaluronic Acid: While often associated with hydration, hyaluronic acid also plays a role in maintaining skin suppleness. It attracts and retains moisture, contributing to a plumper and more youthful complexion.

Sunscreen: Sun protection is a nonnegotiable aspect of any antiaging routine. UV rays contribute significantly to premature aging, causing wrinkles, sunspots, and loss of skin elasticity. Choose a broadspectrum sunscreen with at least SPF 30 and apply it every morning, even on cloudy days.

Eye Creams: The skin around the eyes is delicate and prone to early signs of aging. Eye creams with ingredients like retinol, hyaluronic acid, and peptides can target fine lines, puffiness, and dark circles.

Establishing a Morning skin-care Routine

1. The Morning skin-care Ritual: A Fresh Start:

Your morning skin-care routine sets the tone for the day, providing essential nourishment, protection, and preparation for any makeup application. Establishing a thoughtful morning routine ensures that your skin is equipped to face environmental stressors and maintains its vitality throughout the day.

2. Cleansing: The WakeUp Call for Your Skin:

Cleansing in the morning is crucial to remove any impurities, excess oils, and product residue that may have accumulated overnight. Use a gentle, hydrating cleanser that respects your skin's natural barrier. Avoid harsh cleansers that can strip the skin of its essential oils.

How to Cleanse:

1. Wet your face with lukewarm water.
2. Apply a small amount of cleanser to your fingertips.
3. Gently massage the cleanser onto your face using circular motions.
4. Rinse thoroughly with water and pat your skin dry.

3. Toning: Preparing the Canvas:

Toning is a crucial step that helps balance the skin's pH, remove any remaining traces of impurities, and prepare the skin for subsequent products. Choose a toner that suits your skin type—hydrating toners for dry skin, exfoliating toners for oily skin, and soothing toners for sensitive skin.

How to Tone:

1. Apply a small amount of toner to a cotton pad or your fingertips.
2. Gently sweep the toner across your face, avoiding the eye area.
3. Allow the toner to absorb into your skin before proceeding to the next step.

4.   Serums and Treatments: Targeted Solutions:

Morning serums and treatments focus on addressing specific concerns or providing added protection. Depending on your skin-care goals, you may incorporate serums with ingredients like vitamin C, hyaluronic acid, or peptides.

How to Apply Serums:

1. Dispense a small amount of serum onto your fingertips.
2. Gently pat or massage the serum onto your face and neck.
3. Allow the serum to absorb before moving to the next step.

5. Moisturizing: Hydration Boost:

Moisturizing in the morning is essential to lock in hydration, create a smooth canvas for makeup application, and reinforce the skin's natural barrier. Choose a lightweight, nongreasy moisturizer suitable for your skin type.

How to Moisturize:

1. Apply a small amount of moisturizer to your face and neck.

2. Massage the moisturizer in upward motions until fully absorbed.

3. Ensure that your moisturizer contains SPF or follow up with a separate sunscreen.

6. Sunscreen: Shielding Your Skin:

Sunscreen is the cornerstone of any morning skin-care routine. It protects your skin from the harmful effects of UV rays, prevents premature aging, and reduces the risk of skin cancer.

How to Apply Sunscreen:

1. Use a broadspectrum sunscreen with at least SPF 30.

2. Apply a generous amount to your face, neck, and any exposed areas.

3. Reapply every two hours, especially if you'll be outdoors.

7. Eye Cream: Brightening and Protecting:

If you use an eye cream as part of your routine, apply it in the morning to address specific concerns around the eyes, such as fine lines, puffiness, or dark circles.

How to Apply Eye Cream:

1. Use a small amount of eye cream on your ring finger.

   2. Gently pat the eye cream around
      the orbital bone, avoiding direct
      contact with the eyes.

8. Makeup Application (Optional):

If you wear makeup, the morning routine provides a smooth canvas for application. Choose makeup products that complement your skin-care routine and avoid ingredients that may be harsh on the skin.

How to Apply Makeup:

   1. Start with a makeup primer if desired.

   2. Apply foundation, concealer, and other makeup products as part of your routine.

Enhancing Your skin-care Experience

1. Consistency is Key:

The effectiveness of any skin-care routine lies in consistency. Make a commitment to follow your morning skin-care routine daily to experience the full benefits of the products you've chosen.

2. Patch Testing: Safety First:

Before incorporating new products into your routine, conduct patch tests to ensure compatibility with your skin. Apply a small amount of the product to a discreet area and monitor for any adverse reactions.

3. Understanding Product Interactions:

Some skin-care ingredients may interact negatively with others. For example, using retinoids and vitamin C together may increase the risk of irritation.

Familiarize yourself with potential interactions to maximize the benefits of your chosen products.

4. Adapting to Seasonal Changes:

Your skin's needs may vary with the seasons. Adjust your skin-care routine to accommodate changes in humidity, temperature, and environmental factors. Consider using richer moisturizers in colder months and adapting your sunscreen to higher SPF during sunny seasons.

5. Listening to Your Skin:

Pay attention to how your skin responds to different products and adjust your routine accordingly. If you notice signs of sensitivity or if a product is not delivering the desired results, reassess and make informed adjustments.

6. **Seeking Professional Guidance:**

While upgrading your skin-care routine is a gratifying process, seeking professional guidance can provide invaluable insights. Dermatologists and skin-care professionals can offer personalized recommendations based on your unique skin type, concerns, and goals.

Chapter 6: The Role of Sleep Positions

Impact on Skin Health

The position in which you sleep plays a crucial role in the overall health and appearance of your skin. As you embark on a journey to understand the impact of sleep positions, it becomes evident that nighttime habits extend beyond mere comfort and restfulness—they directly influence the messages conveyed by your morning pillow prints.

1. Pressure Points and Imprints:

Different sleep positions exert varying pressure on specific areas of your face. Side sleepers, for instance, often wake up with imprints on one side, where the face has been pressed against the pillow for an extended period. These imprints may contribute to the development of fine lines and wrinkles, emphasizing the need for strategic position choices to mitigate pressure points.

2. Promotion of Blood Circulation:

The right sleep position can promote optimal blood circulation, contributing to a healthier complexion. Sleeping on your back, also known as the supine position, allows for unrestricted blood flow to the face. Improved circulation facilitates the delivery of oxygen and nutrients to skin cells, promoting a radiant and revitalized complexion.

3. Minimization of Acne and Irritation:

Certain sleep positions can minimize the risk of acne and skin irritation. Back sleeping, in particular, reduces the likelihood of the face coming into contact with bacterialaden pillows, decreasing the chances of breakouts. For individuals prone to acne or skin sensitivity, choosing a sleep position that minimizes facial contact with the pillowcase is a strategic move.

4. Impact on Facial Edema:

Sleep positions influence the distribution of fluids in the facial tissues. Side and stomach sleepers may wake up with more pronounced facial edema due to gravitational effects, leading to puffiness around the eyes and cheeks. This emphasizes the importance of considering your sleep position in managing morning pillow prints and maintaining a more refreshed morning appearance.

Recommended Sleep Positions

Armed with the understanding of the impact of sleep positions on skin health, it's time to explore recommended positions that align with the goal of promoting optimal skin wellbeing. Making intentional choices about your sleep position contributes not only to a more comfortable night's rest but also to waking up with skin that reflects vitality and resilience.

1. Back Sleeping:

Sleeping on your back is widely regarded as one of the best positions for skin health. This position minimizes pressure points, reduces the risk of facial creases, and promotes even blood circulation. Back sleeping is particularly beneficial for individuals prone to acne, as it limits contact between the face and pillow, reducing the transfer of oils and bacteria.

2. Use of Silk or Satin Pillowcases: Regardless of your preferred sleep position, opting for silk or satin pillowcases can benefit your skin. These smooth and gentle fabrics create less friction compared to traditional cotton, reducing the likelihood of pillow-induced imprints and minimizing stress on the skin. Silk and satin also contribute to maintaining the moisture balance of your skin, preventing dehydration.

3. Avoiding Stomach Sleeping:

While stomach sleeping may be comfortable for some, it can contribute to the development of morning pillow prints and facial imprints. The pressure exerted on the face during stomach sleeping may lead to lines and wrinkles over time. If you find it challenging to switch to back sleeping, consider using additional pillows to elevate your head slightly, reducing pressure on the facial skin.

4. Pillow Support for Side Sleepers:

For those who prefer side sleeping, strategic pillow placement can help minimize the impact on facial skin. Place a soft pillow between your knees to align your spine and reduce pressure on the hips. Additionally, consider using a contoured or memory foam pillow that supports the natural curve of your neck, minimizing strain and potential creases.

5. Changing Positions Gradually:

Changing sleep positions may not happen overnight, and it's essential to make adjustments gradually. Begin by incorporating small changes into your routine, such as adding a pillow for support or experimenting with a new sleep position for short durations. This gradual approach allows your body to adapt more comfortably to the desired position.

Understanding the role of sleep positions in the health of your skin empowers you to make intentional choices that align with your skin-care goals. As you embark on the journey to optimize your sleep position, remember that consistency is key. Over time, the benefits of strategic sleep positioning will not only reflect in the mirror each morning but contribute to a holistic approach to skin health.

Chapter 7: Investing in Quality Bedding

Pillow and Bedding Materials

The relationship between your skin and bedding is an intimate one that can significantly impact the health and appearance of your complexion. As we delve into the importance of investing in quality bedding, we focus on two key aspects: pillow and bedding materials.

Pillow Materials:

The material of your pillow can have a profound effect on your skin, especially considering the extended hours spent in direct contact with it. Opting for highquality materials enhances comfort while minimizing the risk of morning pillow prints and potential skin issues.

1. Memory Foam:

Memory foam pillows contour to the shape of your head and neck, providing support and reducing pressure points. This can be particularly beneficial for those prone to waking up with imprints on their faces. The even distribution of weight on a memory foam pillow minimizes the risk of fine lines and wrinkles caused by uneven pressure.

2. Feather and Down:

Feather and down pillows offer a luxurious feel, but their softness may contribute to facial compression and imprints. To mitigate this, consider using a pillow insert with a combination of feathers and down rather than a pillow made entirely from these materials. Additionally, ensure that the pillowcase is made from smooth and breathable fabric.

3. Silk or Satin Pillowcases:

Investing in silk or satin pillowcases is a gamechanger for skin health. These materials create less friction compared to traditional cotton, reducing the likelihood of morning pillow prints and minimizing stress on the skin. Silk and satin also contribute to maintaining the moisture balance of your skin, preventing dehydration.

Bedding Materials:

The material of your sheets and duvet covers plays a crucial role in maintaining skin health. The right bedding materials not only contribute to a restful night's sleep but also create an environment that supports the vitality and resilience of your skin.

1. Cotton:

High-quality, breathable cotton is a popular choice for bedding. It allows for proper airflow, keeping your skin cool and reducing the risk of overheating during the night. Opt for a higher thread count for a smoother and softer feel against your skin. Cotton also absorbs moisture, helping to prevent skin irritation.

2. Bamboo:

Bamboo sheets are prized for their softness and hypoallergenic properties. The natural breathability of bamboo fabric ensures proper ventilation, reducing the risk of sweating and discomfort. Bamboo is also known for its moisture-wicking capabilities, making it an excellent choice for individuals with sensitive or acneprone skin.

3. Micro-fiber:

Micro-fiber sheets are another alternative known for their softness and durability. While they may not be as breathable as natural fibers like cotton or bamboo, microfiber sheets are often more affordable and resistant to wrinkles. Consider the specific needs of your skin and personal preferences when choosing bedding materials.

How Bedding Affects Your Skin

The impact of bedding on your skin goes beyond mere comfort—it directly influences the health and appearance of your complexion. Understanding how bedding affects your skin allows you to make informed choices that contribute to a supportive and nurturing sleep environment.

1. Friction and Pillow Prints:

The friction between your skin and the pillowcase can contribute to the formation of morning pillow prints. Rough or coarse materials may increase friction, leading to more pronounced lines and imprints. Silk or satin pillowcases, with their smooth texture, reduce friction and create a gentler surface for your skin.

2. Breathability and Overheating:

Bedding materials play a role in the breathability of your sleep environment. Proper airflow is essential for preventing overheating, which can lead to increased sweat production and potential skin irritation. Breathable materials like cotton and bamboo promote ventilation, ensuring a comfortable temperature for your skin throughout the night.

3. Moisture Absorption:

The ability of bedding materials to absorb moisture is crucial for maintaining skin health. Excess moisture on the skin can contribute to conditions like acne and irritation. Cotton and bamboo are excellent choices as they absorb moisture, keeping your skin dry and reducing the risk of skin issues.

4. Hypoallergenic Properties:

Bedding materials with hypoallergenic properties are especially beneficial for individuals with sensitive skin or allergies. Bamboo, for example, naturally repels allergens and bacteria. Choosing hypoallergenic materials minimizes the risk of skin reactions and ensures a more comfortable sleep experience.

5. Maintenance and Cleanliness:

The cleanliness of your bedding also directly affects your skin. Dust mites, allergens, and bacteria can accumulate over time, potentially leading to skin issues. Regularly washing and maintaining your bedding, including pillowcases, sheets, and duvet covers, is essential for creating a hygienic sleep environment that supports skin health.

6. Preventing Acne and Irritation:

Bedding materials can contribute to or mitigate the risk of acne and skin irritation. Smooth, breathable fabrics like silk and satin reduce the likelihood of frictioninduced acne and minimize the impact of pressure points on the skin. Choosing bedding materials that align with your skin's needs helps prevent common skin-care concerns.

Investing in quality bedding is an investment in the overall wellbeing of your skin. The thoughtful selection of pillow and bedding materials, considering factors such as friction, breathability, moisture absorption, and cleanliness, contributes to a sleep environment that supports healthy and radiant skin. As you optimize your bedding choices, you create a nurturing space that enhances the symbiotic relationship between your skin and the rejuvenating powers of a good night's sleep.

Chapter 8: Lifestyle Changes for Healthy Skin

Hydration Habits

Healthy, radiant skin often begins from within, and one of the most foundational lifestyle changes you can make is adopting hydration habits that support optimal skin health. Water is not just a vital component for overall wellbeing; it plays a crucial role in the appearance and resilience of your skin. In this chapter, we'll delve into the importance of hydration and practical habits to ensure your skin stays nourished from the inside out.

1. The Role of Hydration in Skin Health:

Adequate hydration is like a daily elixir for your skin. Water plays a pivotal role in maintaining the skin's natural moisture balance, preventing dehydration, and supporting overall skin function. When your body is wellhydrated, your skin is more likely to appear plump, supple, and less prone to fine lines and wrinkles.

2. Daily Water Intake Goals:

The recommended daily water intake varies for each individual based on factors such as age, weight, and activity level. As a general guideline, aim for at least eight 8ounce glasses of water per day, commonly known as the "8x8 rule." However, individual needs may differ, and factors like climate, physical activity, and personal health conditions can influence your water requirements. Pay attention to your body's signals and adjust your water intake accordingly.

3. Incorporating Hydrating Foods:
Hydration isn't solely about the water you drink; it also involves incorporating hydrating foods into your diet. Fruits and vegetables with high water content, such as watermelon, cucumber, oranges, and celery, contribute to your overall hydration levels. Including these foods not only enhances your skin's moisture but also provides essential vitamins and antioxidants that promote skin health.

4. Hydrating Beverages Beyond Water:
While water is the primary source of hydration, incorporating other beverages can contribute to your overall

fluid intake. Herbal teas, infused water with fruits and herbs, and coconut water are excellent options that not only provide hydration but also offer additional benefits. Be mindful of sugary and caffeinated beverages, as excessive consumption can have dehydrating effects.

5. Consistent Hydration Throughout the Day:

The key to maintaining optimal hydration is consistency. Instead of consuming large amounts of water at once, aim for a steady intake throughout the day. Carry a reusable water bottle to encourage regular sips, especially in the morning and afternoon when hydration is crucial for skin health.

6. Monitoring Skin Hydration:

Your skin can provide valuable insights into your hydration levels. If you notice dryness, flakiness, or a lack of skin elasticity, it may be an indication that you need to increase your water intake. Conversely, wellhydrated skin tends to have a more vibrant and plump appearance. Use your skin's condition as a visual guide to adjust your hydration habits.

7. Humidification in Dry Environments:

In dry climates or during the winter months when indoor heating systems can deplete moisture from the air, consider using a humidifier. Humidification helps maintain the skin's hydration levels by preventing excessive water loss. This is particularly beneficial for those with dry or sensitive skin.

Nutritional Considerations

Nutrition is a powerful determinant of skin health. What you consume directly impacts the vitality, resilience, and appearance of your skin. Making thoughtful nutritional choices is an essential lifestyle change that supports healthy skin from the inside. In this section, we'll explore key nutritional considerations and how they contribute to radiant and nourished skin.

1. Anti-oxidantRich Foods:

Anti-oxidants are superheroes for your skin, protecting it from free radical damage caused by environmental factors such as pollution and UV rays. Incorporate a variety of antioxidantrich foods into your diet, including berries, leafy greens, citrus fruits, nuts, and seeds. These foods provide essential vitamins like vitamin C and E, which play a crucial role in skin health.

2. Omega-3 Fatty Acids:

Omega-3 fatty acids are essential for maintaining the skin's natural barrier function. They contribute to skin hydration, reduce inflammation, and support overall skin health. Include sources of omega-3 fatty acids in your diet, such as fatty fish (salmon, mackerel), flaxseeds, chia seeds, and walnuts.

3. Hydration from Within:

While external hydration is vital, nourishing your skin from within is equally important. Waterrich fruits and vegetables, as mentioned earlier, contribute to both hydration and nutritional intake. Cucumbers, watermelon, and oranges, for example, not only provide hydration but also deliver vitamins and minerals essential for skin health.

4. Collagen-Boosting Foods:

Collagen is a structural protein that contributes to the elasticity and firmness of the skin. Including collagenboosting foods in your diet supports the body's natural collagen production. Bone broth, fish, lean meats, and collagenrich vegetables like bell peppers and tomatoes are excellent choices for promoting skin elasticity.

5. Limiting Processed and Sugary Foods:

Processed and sugary foods can contribute to inflammation and skin issues. Highglycemic foods, such as refined carbohydrates and sugary snacks, may exacerbate acne and lead to premature aging. Opt for whole, unprocessed foods, and be mindful of your sugar intake to maintain skin health.

6. Vitamins and Minerals:

Essential vitamins and minerals play diverse roles in skin health. Vitamin A supports cell turnover, vitamin E provides antioxidant protection, and minerals like zinc contribute to wound healing and immune function. Ensure a balanced diet that includes a variety of colorful fruits and vegetables to obtain a spectrum of vitamins and minerals beneficial for your skin.

7. Protein for Skin Repair:

Protein is crucial for skin repair and regeneration. Include lean sources of protein in your diet, such as poultry, fish, tofu, beans, and legumes. Adequate protein intake supports the production of collagen and elastin, contributing to the overall structure and resilience of your skin.

8. Herbal Teas and Green Tea:

Herbal teas and green tea are not only hydrating but also provide additional skin benefits. Green tea, in particular, is rich in antioxidants, including catechins, which have antiinflammatory and protective effects on the skin. Choose unsweetened varieties to maximize their benefits.

9. Moderation and Individualized Choices:

Individual nutritional needs vary, and there is no one-size-fits-all approach to skin-care through diet. Consider factors such as allergies, intolerances, and personal preferences when making nutritional choices. Moderation and balance are key principles for sustaining a diet that supports healthy and radiant skin.

Adopting hydration habits and making thoughtful nutritional considerations are transformative lifestyle changes that contribute to the overall health and vibrancy of your skin. As you integrate these practices into your daily life, you create a foundation for radiant skin from the inside out. In the upcoming chapters, we will continue to explore strategies and insights that enhance your skin-care routine, fostering a holistic approach to skin health.

Chapter 9: DIY Remedies for Pillow Prints

Natural Remedies

Morning pillow prints, those subtle imprints left on your face after a night's sleep, can sometimes leave you wishing for a quick solution to restore your skin's natural vibrancy. In this chapter, we will explore a range of natural remedies that you can easily incorporate into your skin-care routine. These DIY solutions harness the power of natural ingredients and practices to minimize the impact of pillow prints and promote healthier, more radiant skin.

1. Cucumber Slices:

Cucumber slices are a classic remedy for reducing puffiness and soothing the skin. Place chilled cucumber slices on your face, focusing on areas with visible pillow prints. The cool temperature and hydrating properties of cucumbers help constrict blood vessels, reducing inflammation and promoting skin recovery.

How to Use:

1. Slice a cucumber and chill the slices in the refrigerator.
2. Place the chilled cucumber slices on your face, focusing on areas with pillow prints.
3. Leave them on for 10-15 minutes.
4. Gently massage the skin to enhance circulation before rinsing with cool water.

2. Aloe Vera Gel:

Aloe vera is renowned for its soothing and hydrating properties. Applying pure aloe vera gel to your skin can help alleviate irritation and promote skin healing. Aloe vera contains compounds that reduce inflammation, making it an effective natural remedy for addressing morning pillow prints.

How to Use:

1. Extract fresh aloe vera gel from an aloe leaf or use commercially available pure aloe vera gel.
2. Apply a thin layer of the gel to the areas with pillow prints.
3. Leave it on for 15-20 minutes.
4. Rinse with cool water and pat your skin dry.

3. Green Tea Compress:

Green tea is rich in antioxidants and antiinflammatory properties, making it a valuable ingredient for soothing the skin. Create a green tea compress to reduce puffiness and minimize the appearance of pillow prints.

How to Use:

1. Steep two green tea bags in hot water and let them cool.
2. Place the cooled tea bags on your face, concentrating on areas with pillow prints.
3. Leave them on for 10-15 minutes.
4. Gently massage the skin and rinse with cool water.

4. Honey and Yogurt Mask:

Honey is known for its moisturizing and antibacterial properties, while yogurt contains lactic acid, which promotes gentle exfoliation. Combining these ingredients in a mask can help hydrate the skin, reduce the appearance of lines, and enhance overall skin texture.

How to Use:

1. Mix equal parts honey and plain yogurt to form a smooth paste.
2. Apply the mixture to your face, paying attention to areas with pillow prints.
3. Allow it to sit for 15-20 minutes.
4. Rinse off with lukewarm water and pat your skin dry.

5. Rosewater Toner:

Rosewater is a gentle and fragrant solution that helps soothe the skin while maintaining its pH balance. Using rosewater as a toner can refresh your skin, making it a beneficial addition to your morning skin-care routine.

How to Use:

1. Spritz rose-water directly onto your face or apply it with a cotton pad.

2. Use the toner after cleansing your face and before applying moisturizer.

3. Allow it to air dry or gently pat your skin.

6. Ice Roller Massage:

A simple ice roller can work wonders in reducing puffiness and tightening the skin. The cold temperature helps constrict blood vessels, diminishing the appearance of morning pillow prints.

How to Use:

1. Place your ice roller in the freezer for at least a few hours.

2. Roll the chilled ice roller over your face, focusing on areas with pillow prints.

3. Use gentle, upward strokes for a soothing massage.

4. Continue for 5-10 minutes.

7. Oat-meal Scrub:

Oatmeal is a gentle exfoliant that can help remove dead skin cells and promote a smoother complexion. Creating an oatmeal scrub allows you to gently massage the skin, reducing the visibility of pillow prints.

How to Use:

1. Mix ground oats with a small amount of water to create a paste.

2. Apply the oatmeal scrub to your face, focusing on areas with pillow prints.

3. Gently massage in circular motions for 23 minutes.

4. Rinse with lukewarm water and pat your skin dry.

Facial Exercises

Beyond topical remedies, incorporating facial exercises into your routine can strengthen the muscles, improve circulation, and contribute to a more toned and resilient complexion. These DIY facial exercises target areas prone to pillow prints, providing a natural and effective way to enhance your skin's appearance.

1. Cheek Smiling Exercise:

This exercise targets the muscles in your cheeks, helping to lift and tone the skin in that area.

How to Do:

1. Smile widely, exposing your teeth.

2. Hold the smile for 10 seconds.

3. Relax and repeat 10 times.

2. Forehead Smoothing Exercise:

This exercise focuses on reducing lines on the forehead and promoting a smoother appearance.

How to Do:

1. Place your fingertips on your forehead.

2. Gently smooth your fingers outward, applying light pressure.

3. Repeat this motion across your entire forehead for 23 minutes.

3. Jawline Toning Exercise:

Strengthening the muscles along the jawline can contribute to a more defined and uplifted jaw area.

How to Do:

1. Tilt your head back slightly.

2. Jut your lower jaw forward and upward.

3. Hold for 10 seconds and repeat 10 times.

4. Eye Area Massage:

Massaging the eye area helps improve circulation and reduce puffiness, addressing pillow prints around the eyes.

How to Do:

1. Use your ring fingers to gently massage the eye area in circular motions.

2. Start from the inner corners and move outward.

3. Repeat for 23 minutes, focusing on areas with pillow prints.

5. Neck and Chin Toning Exercise:

This exercise targets the neck and chin area, promoting muscle tone and reducing the appearance of lines.

How to Do:

1. Tilt your head back and look toward the ceiling.

2. Pucker your lips as if you're trying to kiss the ceiling.

3. Hold for 5 seconds and repeat 10 times.

6. Lip and Cheek Resilience Exercise:

Enhance the resilience of your lips and cheeks with this simple exercise.

How to Do:

1. Puff your cheeks with air.

2. Transfer the air from one cheek to the other.

3. Repeat this motion for 12 minutes.

7. Overall Face Relaxation:

Relaxing the facial muscles is as important as toning them. This exercise helps release tension and promotes a more serene appearance.

How to Do:

1. Close your eyes and take a deep breath.

2. Exhale slowly, letting go of any tension in your face.

3. Repeat for 5-10 minutes, incorporating mindfulness into the exercise.

Integrating DIY Remedies into Your Routine

To maximize the effectiveness of these DIY remedies, consider integrating them into your skin-care routine in a way that complements your overall approach to skin health. Here's a suggested routine: Morning Routine:

1. Cucumber Slices or Green Tea Compress: Begin your morning routine by placing chilled cucumber slices or green tea bags on areas with visible pillow prints. This reduces puffiness and prepares your skin for the day ahead.

2. Rosewater Toner: After cleansing your face, use rosewater as a toner. This refreshes your skin and provides a hydrating base for subsequent steps.

3. Aloe Vera Gel: Apply pure aloe vera gel to soothe the skin. This step helps address any irritation caused by pillow prints.

4. Sunscreen: Finish your morning routine with a broadspectrum sunscreen to protect your skin from UV rays, especially if you'll be spending time outdoors.

Evening Routine:

1. Oatmeal Scrub (12 times a week): Incorporate the oatmeal scrub into your evening routine 12 times a week to exfoliate the skin and promote a smoother complexion.

2. Honey and Yogurt Mask (12 times a week): Apply the honey and yogurt mask 12 times a week for added hydration and to improve overall skin texture.

3. Facial Exercises: Dedicate a few minutes to facial exercises in the evening, targeting areas prone to pillow prints. This enhances muscle tone and circulation.

4. Moisturizer: Conclude your evening routine with a moisturizer suitable for your skin type to maintain hydration overnight.

Consistency and Observations

Consistency is key when incorporating DIY remedies into your skin-care routine. Monitor your skin's response to these remedies and exercises over time. Keep a skin-care journal to track any changes in the appearance of pillow prints, skin texture, and overall skin health. Adjust your routine based on your observations, tailoring it to the evolving needs of your skin.

By integrating natural remedies and facial exercises into your skin-care routine, you empower yourself with simple yet effective tools to address morning pillow prints and promote the health and radiance of your skin. As we continue our exploration in the following chapters, we will delve into additional strategies to enhance your skin-care journey, fostering a holistic approach to skin wellbeing.

Chapter 10: Consultation with skin-care Professionals

Skin-care is a deeply personal journey, and while DIY remedies and athome practices can be beneficial, there comes a point when seeking guidance from skin-care professionals becomes a valuable step in achieving optimal skin health. In this chapter, we will explore the significance of consulting with skin-care professionals, focusing on dermatologist visits and the creation of customized skin-care plans. These expert-led approaches are designed to address individual skin concerns, provide targeted solutions, and elevate your skin-care routine to new heights.

Dermatologist Visits

1.   **Understanding the Role of Dermatologists:**

Dermatologists are medical professionals who specialize in the diagnosis and treatment of conditions related to the skin, hair, and nails. Consulting with a dermatologist goes beyond addressing cosmetic concerns; it encompasses the evaluation and management of various skin health issues, ranging from medical conditions to aesthetic goals.

2.   **When to Consider a Dermatologist Visit:**

While many skin-care concerns can be managed with over-the-counter products and lifestyle adjustments, certain signs and symptoms warrant the expertise of a dermatologist. Consider scheduling a dermatologist visit if you experience:

1. Persistent acne or breakouts that don't respond to over-the-counter treatments.

2. Skin conditions such as eczema, psoriasis, or rosacea.

3. Suspicious moles or changes in existing moles that may indicate skin cancer.

4. Chronic skin issues such as persistent dryness, redness, or itching.

5. Signs of premature aging, including fine lines, wrinkles, and sun damage.

6. Hair loss or scalp conditions that require specialized attention.

7. Any sudden or concerning changes in the appearance of your skin.

3. The Dermatologist Consultation Process:

A dermatologist consultation typically involves a thorough examination of your skin, discussion of your medical history, and an exploration of your specific concerns and goals. The process may include:

Skin Examination: The dermatologist will visually inspect your skin, identifying any areas of concern, moles, or abnormalities. They may use specialized tools, such as a dermatoscope, to closely examine specific areas.

Medical History: Providing information about your medical history, including previous skin conditions, allergies, medications, and lifestyle factors, helps the dermatologist gain a comprehensive understanding of your skin health.

Discussion of Concerns: Communicate openly about your skin-care concerns, whether they are related to medical conditions, cosmetic goals, or both. Clear communication enables the dermatologist to tailor their recommendations to your individual needs.

Diagnostic Tests: In some cases, the dermatologist may recommend diagnostic tests, such as skin biopsies or patch tests, to gather more information about your skin's condition.

4. Treatment Options and Recommendations:

Based on the evaluation, the dermatologist will discuss potential treatment options and recommend a personalized skin-care plan. This plan may include:

Prescription Medications: For certain skin conditions, dermatologists may prescribe topical or oral medications to address underlying issues and promote healing.

In-office Procedures: Dermatologists offer a range of in-office procedures for both medical and cosmetic purposes. These may include laser treatments, chemical peels, injectables, and surgical procedures.

Skin-care Recommendations: Dermatologists can provide tailored recommendations for skin-care products based on your skin type, concerns, and any specific conditions you may have.

Sun Protection Guidance: Sun protection is a cornerstone of skin-care. Dermatologists emphasize the importance of using sunscreen daily and may recommend specific products suited to your skin type.

5. Followup Visits and Monitoring:

Dermatologist visits are often part of an ongoing relationship aimed at maintaining and optimizing your skin health. Followup visits allow the dermatologist to monitor your progress, adjust treatment plans if necessary, and address any new concerns that may arise.

Customized skin-care Plans

1. The Need for Customization:

Every individual's skin is unique, influenced by genetics, lifestyle, environmental factors, and specific concerns. A one-size-fits-all approach to skin-care may not address the nuances of individual skin types and conditions. Customized skin-care plans, often created in collaboration with skin-care professionals, recognize the importance of tailoring routines to meet the specific needs of each person.

2. Working with skin-care Professionals for Customization:

skin-care professionals, including dermatologists and licensed aestheticians, play a crucial role in creating personalized skin-care plans. Their expertise allows them to assess your skin's current state, identify specific concerns, and recommend targeted solutions. The collaborative nature of working with skin-care professionals ensures that your skin-care plan aligns with both your goals and the unique characteristics of your skin.

3. Key Components of Customized skin-care Plans:

A customized skin-care plan typically includes the following components:

Cleansing Routine: Tailored recommendations for cleansers based on your skin type and concerns.

Treatment Products: Specific treatments such as serums, acids, or retinoids to address concerns like acne, hyperpigmentation, or signs of aging.

Moisturizers: Recommendations for moisturizers that provide the right balance of hydration without causing irritation.

Sunscreen: A crucial component of any skin-care plan, with guidance on selecting a sunscreen that suits your skin type and provides adequate protection.

Specialized Products: If you have specific concerns, such as sensitivity or conditions like rosacea, the skin-care plan may include specialized products to address these issues.

In-office Procedures: For individuals seeking more advanced solutions, the skin-care plan may integrate in-office procedures recommended by skin-care professionals.

4. Adjustments Over Time:

The dynamic nature of skin means that its needs may change over time. Customized skin-care plans are designed to evolve along with your skin. Regular checkins with skin-care professionals allow for adjustments based on changes in your skin health, lifestyle, or treatment goals.

5. Educational Component:

An essential aspect of customized skin-care plans is education. skin-care professionals guide you on how to use products effectively, explain the purpose of each product, and provide insights into maintaining healthy skin-care habits. This knowledge empowers you to take an active role in your skin-care journey.

6. Integration with Lifestyle Choices:

Customized skin-care plans take into account lifestyle factors that can impact skin health. skin-care professionals may offer guidance on factors such as diet, stress management, and sleep, recognizing their role in overall skin wellbeing.

7. Holistic Approach:

The customization process embraces a holistic approach to skin-care. It considers not only individual skin concerns but also the interconnected aspects of wellbeing that contribute to healthy, radiant skin.

Empowering Your skin-care Journey

Consulting with skin-care professionals and embracing customized skin-care plans empowers you with expert guidance and targeted solutions for your skin. By doing so, you align your skin-care routine with evidencebased practices, ensuring that your efforts yield meaningful and lasting results.

Whether you're seeking the expertise of a dermatologist for medical concerns or collaborating with skin-care professionals for a personalized skin-care plan, the journey toward optimal skin health becomes a partnership. skin-care professionals bring a wealth of knowledge, experience, and resources to the table, guiding you on a path that addresses your unique needs and cultivates a foundation for lifelong skin wellbeing.